7 STEPS
TO HEAL SIBO

Simple strategies and exercises
to understand SIBO,
restore energy, beat belly fat
and eliminate brain fog

GRACE LIU, PHARMD

TABLE OF CONTENTS

Foreword: Health is Everything 05

Introducing SIBO & How it Affects Your Health 09

Reviving Bacteria Through Ancient Grains 21

Adding Good Bacteria Back to the Gut with Probiotics 31

Fueling Your Bacteria with Bionic Fiber 43

Stepping Your Way to a Healthier Gut 51

Preventing Leaky Gut By Avoiding Toxic Foods 57

Solidifying a Healthy Gut By Reducing Stress 69

References 79

FOREWORD

Health is Everything

— BY KYLE GRAY

Health is everything.

It's the foundation for everything else in your life.

Friends and family are important, but if you don't have health, it's hard to be there for them.

Love is important, but losing health can test the limits of even the strongest relationships.

Intelligence and positive thinking are important, but it's very difficult to keep a good mindset when your biology is out of balance.

Money is important, but there's no price too high when it comes to your health.

Health is everything.

This, unfortunately, seems to be a lesson most of us need to learn the hard way. I certainly did.

It's graduation day, a day that should be one of the happiest of my life. I've just completed my Master's degree, a proud day made even prouder by the fact that I graduated debt-free and paid for it myself.

They call my name and I'm walking across the stage in front of my family and hundreds of others, my big gown masking a subtle limp. I make my best effort to bring a smile to my face, but it comes out a little crooked.

I'm here to celebrate the achievements of my mind, but I can't help but feel betrayed by my body. My jaw feels like it's about to fall off my face, I have to be careful with what I chew to not spark nasty headaches and I fear going to sleep at night and grinding my teeth. I fear starting my day each morning wondering if I am going to "freak out" with a spontaneous anxiety attack. I can't hike more than a quarter mile without some serious knee pain, and as someone who loves being outdoors, this feels like a prison sentence. Somehow this does not feel like the basic "just getting older" or "overworked student" kind of stuff.

I started visiting various doctors, dentists, chiropractors and other health professionals to help. I sank thousands and thousands of dollars into different treatments. Through various tests, I discovered I had a thyroid problem and that this may be the source of much of what I was going through.

So let's dive in.

Over the next few years, I took thyroid supplements and other vitamins to manage things. I was feeling a little better, but I knew I was in a holding pattern. Almost all of the solutions I found seemed to be a "band-aid on a broken bone" type of treatment. Was I just going to have to mask my symptoms for the rest of my life with a bowl full of pills every day?

I had nearly resigned myself to a life of mediocre health, until the day I met Dr. Grace Liu, PharmD. She was different. She had a confidence in her process and my ability to heal that I had never seen in another doctor. Where other doctors sought to treat symptoms, Dr. Grace targeted the root of the problem: my gut health. This was something I had never even considered, nor heard about from any other health professional I had worked with. Yet it was a key factor in my disease, Hashimoto's, and many other common problems, like SIBO.

Where most had a vague and uncertain process, she had a clear roadmap to recover my health. I knew where we were going and what to expect, which can be one of the most comforting and empowering elements of the healing process.

Within a month of beginning to work with Dr. Grace, the anxiety that once plagued me had cleared. After three months, my joint pain faded and I had never felt stronger, more confident and clearer minded in my entire life. Perhaps most importantly, I once again believed in my ability to heal.

If you are reading this, then you or someone you know could probably also use a dose of hope on their healing journey. You've come to the right place. There's no miracles or magic at play here, but if you trust Dr. Grace's process, you may feel like there is. It's not always easy, and it does require some changes in your daily habits, but if you stick with it, the rewards far outweigh the sacrifices required.

I want to congratulate you on your courage to heal yourself and live a life you truly deserve. Though it may not seem like it right now, you're probably closer than you think.

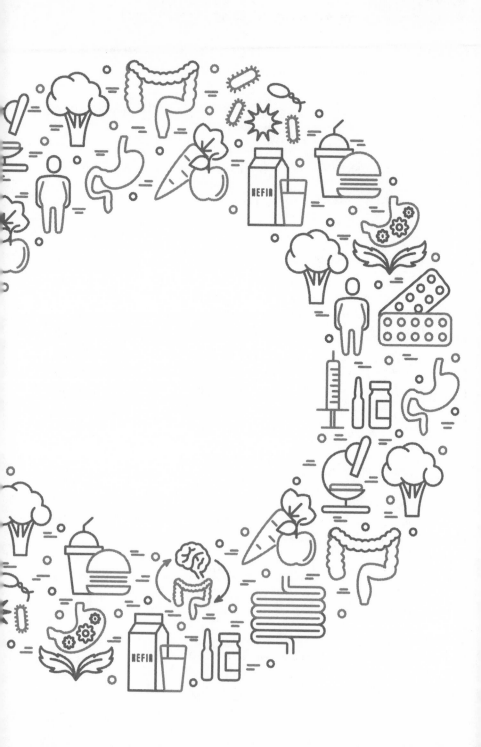

CHAPTER 1

Introducing SIBO & How it Affects Your Health

The gut microbiome is the other side of us. We all have one. In fact, for every one of our cells, there's also a cell from our microbial flora, made up of bacteria, fungi, phages, viruses and sometimes even worms and helminths, which are multicellular eukaryotic organisms. Together, these cells weigh up to 2.5 pounds, which is almost as much as the human brain.

The microbiome is the forgotten organ—we don't even think about it as an organ, but it can get damaged or broken like any other organ can. This is what I help fix at The Gut Institute, my educational platform dedicated to awareness and research about topics related to gut microbiota.

One of the ways the gut can be "damaged" is through imbalances of the microbial flora within us. These types of imbalances cause things like small intestinal bacterial overgrowth, or SIBO (we'll explore what SIBO is soon). SIBO can cause a wide variety of health problems, from immune challenges, to skin disorders, to weight loss.

Fortunately, SIBO is not a permanent problem. All it takes is a few small changes to your diet and lifestyle to achieve a healthier microbiome. I have developed a process of 7 simple steps you can take at home to diminish or reverse the signs of SIBO. Each step is small and easy; you can implement one of them each day.

This process probably isn't going to cure your SIBO in a week, but it can make a big impact and put you on the right path to improving your health and restoring your vitality. What's even better is that all of these steps are inexpensive or free!

For step 1, we need to establish a basic understanding of the symptoms and causes of SIBO, then take a step in the right direction of restoring healthy microbiota by eating fermented foods.

UNDERSTANDING SIBO

Essentially, SIBO refers to the excessive growth of bacteria in the small intestine, which can cause chronic digestive problems as well as many other harmful symptoms.

A close cousin to SIBO is irritable bowel syndrome, or IBS. More severe conditions, such as colitis and inflammatory bowel disease, are also closely linked to SIBO. Yet another condition that you might be familiar with is called SIFO, or small intestinal fungal overgrowth. The major difference between the two is that SIFO is a subclinical fungal infection in the gut, whereas SIBO is a bacterial infection, but many of the symptoms and strategies to treat SIBO are the same because these overgrowths occur simultaneously in 100% of the cases that I have observed.

Bacteria and fungi are totally different life forms. Fungi are actually similar to our cells—fungi, human cells and plant cells are all eukaryotic (meaning they work like animal or plant cells rather than bacteria). However, if there is a bacterial overgrowth, there is inevitably also a fungal overgrowth. This means that when I talk about SIBO, I'm talking about SIFO, too. Therefore, when we are discussing SIBO, what I am referring to is SIBO-SIFO.

It is important to me to be clear about this. There is a "microbial myth" occurring within both the internet and functional medicine worlds that these exist exclusive of each other. Studies show that, after chemical distress or antibiotics, both bacterial and fungal overgrowths occur. The dysbiosis goes deep. Multiple levels of microbial life and kingdoms in our guts become disturbed. Our microbiome is like a rainforest, and after antibiotics or other distressors, the rainforest can become like a barren wasteland. Only the toughest and most tenacious life forms are able to resist being obliterated. These characters are typically the gang leaders, mo'fo Sopranos and Godfathers that take residence, not the angels! Be not afraid. These changes are temporary. With our 7 Steps and The Gut Institute's gut protocols, we can quickly resurrect the protective angels of the microbiome.

SYMPTOMS OF SIBO

So, how can you tell if you have SIBO? The symptoms typically vary from person to person. It depends on your genetics and your toxin burden. In most cases, your symptoms may not seem obviously connected to gut health, but they actually are.

SIBO can cause a variety of symptoms like:

— Bloating
— Vomiting
— Diarrhea

- Weight loss
- Fat gain and the inability to put on lean mass
- Joint pain
- Fibromyalgia
- Chronic fatigue
- Rashes and skin disorders
- Dry spots
- Wrinkles
- Acne
- Atopic dermatitis
- Psoriasis
- Eczema
- Asthma
- Depression
- Poor mood
- Agitation
- Bipolar
- Suicidal thoughts or self harm
- Immune challenges

These conditions are already so bad on their own, but together, they spill into all other areas of your life. They can lead to many other things, like draining your energy, reducing your nutrients and not feeling the same as you did when you were vibrant, healthy and thriving. You might be agitated or depressed and unable to sleep well, or you may feel tired but wired or have a lot of energy at the wrong times. I also think of SIBO as the "gateway gut disorder." If it goes untreated, it can invite worse conditions like autoimmune disorders or even cancer.

All these things are actually related to our gut and the lack of the good bacteria in it. When your gut microbiome is out of balance, you're not absorbing everything you should be from your small intestine. However, because of their singular root cause, all of these symptoms can be cleared up in just two to four weeks—possibly longer, in moderate to severe cases—when the gut is finally addressed.

WHAT CAUSES SIBO?

The causes of SIBO are very clear. In today's world, we are not allied with our bacterial friends and our microflora. We no longer play in the dirt. We eat a standard American diet, which is really refined and has very low fiber, so there are no probiotics or prebiotics—the super fuel that feeds all of our protective allies in the gut.

The common cause of SIBO is antibiotics. On average in the United States, we get 18 to 20 courses of antibiotics before the age of 18. Not only that, but our animals—all our beef, pork and chicken—are also getting a lot of antibiotics. These antibiotics kill off the good and bad bacteria in the gut, opening the door for imbalances. Studies reveal that if a child gets 3 or more courses of antibiotics before age 2, the risk for obesity at age 4 increases by 21%. The more broad-spectrum the strength of the antibiotic, the more likely obesity may occur later in life. It is ironic since antibiotics may help a fever or sniffle, but they appear to set us up for worse infections later. Other studies make clear that our risk for lethal infections such as Clostridium difficile colitis goes up with use of antibiotics. Two courses of antibiotics were associated with more than double the risk of a Clostridium difficile infection later, and 5 courses with 10-fold higher chances.

Parasites are another cause of SIBO. Our western world is not free of parasites. If you don't have the good gut allies, parasites will be free to colonize you. Normally, the gut allies and probiotics can prevent parasites, but a lot of us don't have them because of genetics, toxic burdens and antibiotics.

In the end, it all starts with the gut. People may not feel like they have the signs or symptoms of SIBO, but with special testing like we perform at The Gut Institute, it's very obvious. When we reduce this bacterial growth in the gut, people feel better. All their signs improve, whether it's cancer risk, inflammation, achiness, headaches, fertility issues or fatigue.

You can impact all parts of your body by looking at the gut and SIBO. You don't want to open the door to all the potentially uglier conditions, so you need to start early.

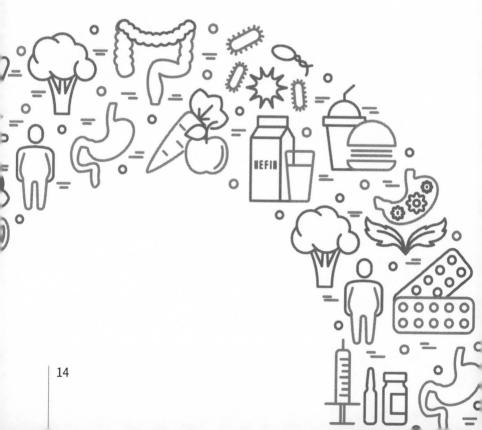

Eating Fermented Foods

All of this brings us to Step 1: fermented foods. In the modern world, everything is refrigerated. We no longer have many foods with probiotics and fiber that really keep our gut healthy. The lifestyle and the things we put in our mouths that can truly reset our gut actually emulate our ancient lives.

BENEFITS OF FERMENTED FOODS

So why do we want to eat fermented foods? Just a few benefits they provide to our gut microbiome include:

— Natural acids
— Healthy gut bacteria
— Digestive enzymes
— Vitamins

One of the best things about fermented food is that it aids and supports our digestion through natural acid. Our gut microbiome loves acidity. In the stomach, our pH goes down to as low as 1 or 2 (the pH scale goes from 1 to 14, with 7 being neutral and 1 being very acidic), so it can kill off any parasites or pathogens in our food, if it happens to have any.

Studies show that as soon as someone takes an acid blocker or proton pump inhibitor (PPI), they immediately get overgrown with pathogenic fungus and bacteria. They are at a higher risk for pneumonia and upper respiratory infections and even deadly Clostridium difficile gut infections. This is because the lack of acidity allows pathogens to proliferate in the whole lung area, which then becomes toxic to the person.

Another benefit of fermentation is the restoration of bacteria in the gut. Our food used to have a lot of dirt on it, so we had natural exposure to all sorts of microbes, good and bad. Nowadays, this exposure is very limited.

Many fermented foods have all the best kinds of bacteria that are components of the natural gut microbiome. These bacteria may be transient, like little travelers that stay for a couple weeks and then go away, or they might be hardcore and stay right at the mucosal lining.

All fermented foods are also rich in enzymes. We may not make all of these enzymes ourselves, but when we eat them, they're bioactive and help to further break down a lot of our foods.

Additionally, fermented foods are rich in vitamins. They contain a lot of folates, as well as B vitamins and many other chemicals that keep us healthy, strong and disease-free, such as fiber and protein. Even if you take the highest-quality vitamins and supplements available, you still might not be absorbing them very well in your gut. This is because we need the bacteria that are often found in fermented foods to help integrate those vitamins into our cells.

COMMON TYPES OF FERMENTED FOODS

You can purchase fermented foods from the store, or you can learn to ferment foods at home on your own. If you have a garden and are overflowing with produce, consider fermenting and storing it.

Here are just a few popular fermented foods you can make or buy:

— Water kefir
— Kombucha
— Kvass
— Kimchi
— Sauerkraut
— Pickles
— Fermented sourdough bread
— Fermented butter
— Yogurt
— Miso
— Natto (fermented soybeans)
— Salami
— Prosciutto

Sourdough bread might be difficult to handle if you have a gluten sensitivity. After our series of 7 Steps, many people find that they can eventually tolerate gluten again, but for now, consider using other ancient grains that are gluten-free to make these types of fermented starches yourself.

Other foods you can think about are cultured, like butter. These kinds of foods are awesome, because you can leave them out on the counter and they won't go bad due to the bacteria that keep them healthy and safe.

If a food is fermented the proper way, it doesn't get moldy because the bacteria that colonize fermented foods are super antifungal. This also means your fermented foods will help battle SIFO, your small intestinal fungal overgrowth.

Not everyone is going to be able to tolerate fermented foods right away because of histamines—chemicals produced during allergy responses. Trying fermented foods is almost a sort of litmus test. If you have really severe SIBO and SIFO, you're probably going to find that the histamines produced by the bacteria in fermented foods will be too much for you.

Ideally, you should not have problems with histamines, no matter what your genetics are, because our ancestors all ate fermented foods. There was no refrigeration, and the foods they ate were either naturally fermented or had to be super fresh. All cultures learned how to ferment foods because that was how they could have sustenance throughout all seasons and not starve to death.

Because of this history, histamines weren't a problem for a lot of people. It's only an issue in the modern day because our gut flora has been affected. After taking antibiotics, we lose the good bacteria that break down histamines for us.

Ultimately, eating fermented food is one of the best things we can do to nourish and fill in all these gaps until the gut is able to do a lot more on its own. I encourage nearly all of my clients to eat fermented foods when it's the appropriate time, and everyone always says that they feel so much better once they can incorporate them into their regular diets and be really healthy.

Taking The First Step
Toward Balance

To kick off your process of rebalancing your gut microbiome and battling SIBO, try a few bites of fermented food every day. You can get really creative and find different things in order to add fermented foods into your diet, but you don't have to go overboard.

Try a little and see how your gut tolerates it. If you experience intolerance, it might be too early for you and you'll need a little more work on your gut before you should try again. But if you do tolerate the fermented food, try eating it a little bit every day and see if you can notice a difference.

Don't forget to take the free 7-day companion course video lessons and check out the extra information at HealSIBO.com.

CHAPTER 2

Reviving Bacteria Through Ancient Grains

Our digestive systems play a larger role in total-body health than we often realize. Within your gut are hundreds of trillions of bacteria, fungi, viruses, phages and more that can influence the way your body functions. Small intestinal bacterial overgrowth, or SIBO, can have major influences on our health. This is why it's so important to overcome it and reset our natural microbiomes.

As part of my 7-Step process to overcome SIBO, you can work to implement certain foods into your diet that can help foster good bacteria and fungi to recreate harmony among your gut flora and cure the nasty symptoms of this imbalance.

ASSESSING YOUR PROGRESS FROM STEP 1

To recap the first step to overcoming SIBO, I suggested that you implement small amounts of fermented foods into your diet. Fermented foods have a significant concentration of good gut bacteria that we don't get much exposure to in our modern era. Additionally, fermented foods can add more natural acids, enzymes and vitamins to your gut to create a healthier ecosystem.

Sometimes, with a new type of food or diet change, the transition may not go super smoothly at first. This can tell you a lot about the current state of your gut—it's like a litmus test for the present gut flora and toxic burden. If you have a severe reaction to fermented foods after trying a few bites—such as a rash, severe diarrhea or constipation—the food is probably a mismatch for your gut. When this occurs, don't continue to eat the food and work on balancing out your gut flora a little more first.

Otherwise, if your gut doesn't feel awful after trying it, then it's a good, smooth transition that can be good for your gut. You should continue eating small amounts of these foods a little longer to see the benefits, and then move on to Step 2.

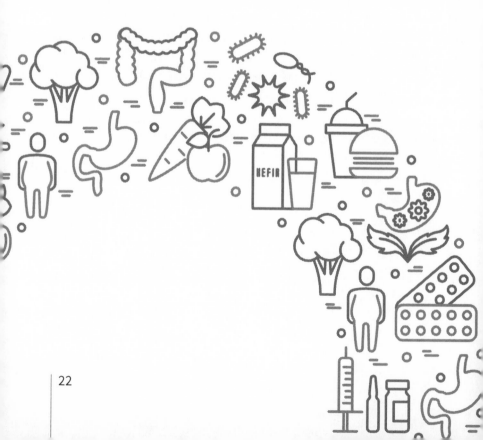

Eating Ancient Grains

Step 2 in our journey to battling SIBO involves cooking and eating ancient grains. These grains contain long chains of glucose, or sugar, that the body uses for energy.

But why would we want to discuss ancient grains when so many people's guts feel better on a keto or a low-carb diet? Many people have trouble breaking down the compounds found in grains and starches, and the reason for this is because they lack a lot of the good bacteria that help with digestion. Antibiotics, in particular, tend to wipe out many forms of these good bacteria, such as the probiotics Bifidobacteria and Lactobacilli, as well as Bacteroidetes and Firmicutes.

You are, yourself, a pharmacy, and the medicine is in your gut and the good flora. These types of bacteria produce protective chemicals for our bodies and aid in breaking down certain types of foods. These chemicals may help prevent inflammation and even cancer.

On the flip side, the bad bacteria produce harmful chemicals from these foods that cause things like body fat, brain fog, mood problems, fatigue and other strange symptoms.

Today, we tend to eat more low-fiber starches or processed grains, which do not contain the same nutrients or fibers that ancient grains do. When we talk about ancient grains and ancient starches, we are referring to whole grains that are less processed or refined, like quinoa or teff. These grains have higher contents of protein, omega-3 fatty acids and fiber.

WHAT ANCIENT GRAINS DO IN THE GUT

Eating ancient grains can be a key strategy that resurrects and repopulates the good bacteria in your gut. This is because ancient grains contain a special kind of fiber that super-feeds the protective allies in your gut mucosal lining.

When ancient grains are cooked, they contain type 3 resistant starch (RS3). Cooking brings out the starches from tight, coiled granules into a gooey gel. Unlike other types of starches, resistant starch resists digestion and, instead, travels to the colon. Aided by the acid in your stomach, this starch becomes something called prebiotic fiber. The prebiotic fiber ferments in the intestines, producing short-chain fatty acids like butyrate, which then feed other helpful bacteria in your colon.

If you have plenty of acidity in your gut, you're maximizing the fiber content found in these ancient grains and starches. Studies show that if you eat plenty of lemon juice or vinegar, like in a salad dressing or naturally fermented foods (pickles, kimchee, sauerkraut), the acidity is chemically modifying the long chains of starch into indigestible fiber. RS3 is resistant to being broken down and digested by our enzymes. RS3 not only lowers the glycemic impact of your foods on blood sugar, but also creates ultra potent fuel for your flora. When your digestive system contains plenty of gastric acid juices, the pH in your stomach is able to lower to 1 or 2, and you'll be able to make more prebiotic fiber. RS3 represents the most resistant starch part of starchy grains, legumes and tubers. To be created, it has be cooked (gelatinized). The more the starch has been processed by either acidifying or reheating, the more

RS3 fuel for the 100 trillion hungry bugs. Humans are the only mammals on Earth to purposefully cook and create culinary masterpieces. Guess what? Boiling and BBQing are likely to be the activities that lead to the evolution of many important things including brains, biomes and taste buds.

TYPES OF ANCIENT GRAINS TO CONSIDER

At this stage in your gut microbiome healing, you should avoid eating gluten-containing starches. Gluten can be very difficult for the digestive system to break down and can cause gut problems, even if you don't have Celiac Disease. For now, stay away from things like wheat (bread, pasta, cookies, cakes), wheat germ, spelt, kamut, einkorn, bulgur, barley, rye and farro.

There are a lot of gluten-free ancient grains that you can eat instead:

— Quinoa
— Teff
— Amaranth
— Brown, black, red and purple rice
— Buckwheat
— Gluten-free oats
— Ancient blue corn
— Millet
— Sorghum

These all contain those resistant starches that turn into prebiotic fiber. Many of these ancient grains contain other good things for us, too. Quinoa, which is actually a seed, happens to have all the amino acids we need and is a complete protein. Dark-colored rices and blue corn contain proanthocyanidins, which are awesome antioxidants.

For a simple recipe, I like to mix a lot of these grains in with white rice, soak them overnight and steam them.

You can also try adding some ancient starches into your diet, such as purple potatoes and other tubers, beans and lentils. These foods have the same kinds of resistant starches that ancient grains do, which will help fuel the bacteria in your gut mucosal lining.

There are many ways to prepare these foods for yourself and your family. For example, purple potatoes can be roasted whole and served with butter and olive oil, or with rosemary and other herbs, salt and lemon. Lentils are great served in soup.

Beans need to be soaked—if you're still committed to fermented foods from Step 1, you can even add a little sauerkraut juice or kimchi juice while they're soaking. These have really high natural *Lactobacilli*, good probiotics which transform the food into a more bioavailable protein source, and a more bioavailable fiber source, as well. A better kind of starch comes out of that. You can even sprout the beans before cooking for more nutrients. My sister Marisa sprouts all her beans. It is an incredible feat that impresses me to no end.

DO ANCIENT GRAINS AFFECT BLOOD SUGAR?

If you have type 2 diabetes or are otherwise concerned about your blood sugar levels, you might be hesitant to add ancient grains to your diet because of the carbohydrates. However, these grains do not always affect blood sugar levels. It really depends on what is growing in your gut—if you have pathogens that are sugar- and carb-eating in there, and how much Bifidobacteria (Bifido) you have.

Ancient grains contain polysaccharides, which are long chains of glucose.

These chains take longer for the body to break down and sugar enters the bloodstream more slowly, which helps blood sugar levels stay more consistent. Additionally, the resistant starches found in ancient grains are not digested at all, meaning they won't affect your blood sugar.

You can also add more acids to your meals to make sure your stomach is prepared to create prebiotic fiber out of the resistant starches you eat, rather than break them down. I sometimes supplement using a tablespoon or two of apple cider vinegar or a tablespoon of lemon juice in my water, or by eating plenty of salad with vinegar on it. A small cup of low-sugar kombucha is fantastic as a digestive tonic with meals for this reason. My favorite brands are High Country from Vail, Colorado and local brands such as Sprouts and Safeway. These are low sugar and contain Acetobacter probiotic for that sublime acid balance. The key here is to mimic a well-functioning gut microbiome until it gets to where we actually need it to be: a healthy, balanced gut.

Eating carbohydrates can also affect some people in other negative ways, causing bloating. People who are missing good Bifido like *Bifidobacteria longum* lack the gut flora needed to break down carbs properly. If bad sugar-eating bacteria and yeasts overtake the intestines, they can pump out chemicals that become toxic to your body. One chemical is called oxalates which can crystallize with calcium and heavy metals and cause nodules, lumps, achy muscles, achy joints and kidney stones. Many probiotic strains such as are inherently capable of neutralizing oxalates for you so they do not become problematic.

Antibiotics can be terrifying for the microbiome because they kill off *Bifidobacteria longum* and other gut guardians which keep you happy and whole. Overcoming SIBO can help you regulate the bad bacteria so eating carbs is less harmful to your health.

"I have experienced many benefits working with Dr. Grace. I only lost 1 pound on the scale, but I lost a very 'puffy' face and regained my old sexy abs. I used to be a fitness competitor. On my last vacation to Europe, for the first time in a long while, I wore a bikini. My sinus congestion is pretty much gone on her protocols. Now I can eat gluten again. Thank you so much, Dr. Grace!"

— **TRISHA W.,** Nevada

Working Toward a Balanced Microbiome

You might be wondering, "If ancient grains are so great, why don't we see a lot of them right now?" This is probably because they're not mass-produced in fields of one product. The grains we tend to eat are more processed and refined, which improves shelf life.

In the beginning, a lot of people won't be able to tolerate a lot of ancient grains or starches. However, you might be shocked to see that just a few bites are tolerable. This is a great way to get the gut flora resurrected again, especially when they're missing after taking antibiotics, enduring high stress or after eating the standard American diet, or a low-fiber diet.

Once people add in ancient grains or other ancient starches like tubers or lentils and beans to their diets, they often find a new degree of health. They are shocked that they can quickly emerge from a specific-carb diet, which is very restrictive for carbs. When they transition, their gut flora helps them maintain their ability to break down starches and integrate them into the body.

Everyone's gut is different, and your microbiome may be more or less balanced than someone else's. This might mean that you are unable to tolerate high amounts of ancient grains and starches right away. You may need to do multiple phases to treat SIBO and SIFO, and in the first phase, it may be more difficult to begin implementing these types of foods.

Even still, I encourage you to take a few bites of ancient grains and starches, even if it's only once every few days. Then, as your gut gets stronger and stronger, you can start to expand from this. The smallest amount can help resurrect your good bacteria and anchor within the gut, promoting future balance and a healthy body.

Don't forget to take the free 7-day companion course video lessons and check out the extra information at HealSIBO.com.

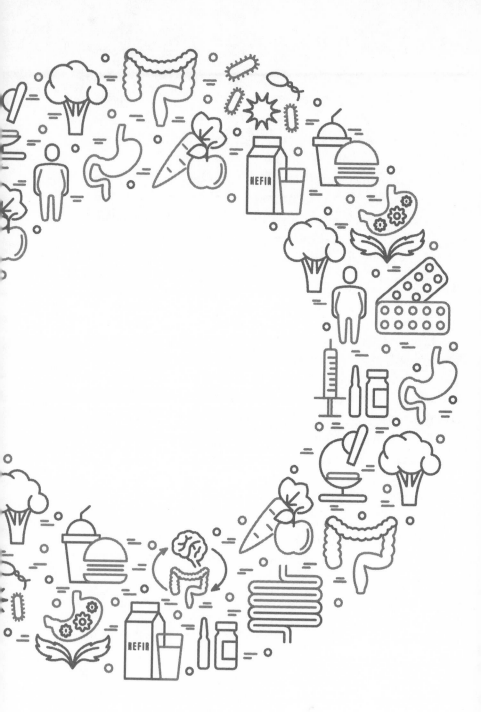

CHAPTER 3

Adding Good Bacteria Back to the Gut with Probiotics

After following the last 2 steps of my 7-step process to overcoming SIBO, or small intestinal bacterial overgrowth, your gut may be experiencing some changes. The good bacteria, enzymes and acids introduced with fermented foods in Step 1 and the prebiotic fiber introduced through ancient grains in Step 2 will be starting to prepare your gut microbiome to allow more of the good guys in—the healthy bacteria that should be in your intestines from the get-go.

Attempting to eat just a few bites of ancient grains or starches every few days can get the bacteria in your gut starting to use that healthy prebiotic fiber. The bacteria that transform prebiotic fiber into short-chain fatty acids, which feed the gut flora in your gut mucosal lining, are actually the same kind found in many probiotics. (I'll explain more about probiotics in a bit.)

If you had trouble with even minor amounts of ancient grains, the addition of probiotics in Step 3 might make it easier for you to eat these types of foods. With this next tip, you'll be introducing more of the good bacteria into your gut that will aid in the breakdown of these healthy fibers and other compounds over time.

Introducing Probiotics — Gut Guardians

Something you might not know about human beings is that, out of all the animals on Earth, we have the least number of flora in the small intestine. There are a couple different theories as to why this is.

One theory is that the complex carbohydrates that were cooked after humans discovered fire really fed our brain, and we got bigger and smarter as a result. After this, we started eating all kinds of foods that really were fueling the size and growth of the human brain, like cooked proteins, cooked starches and fats. In order to absorb all these foods in the small intestine and not create a bunch of bacterial havoc, our small intestine became very sterile, with the benefit of probiotics.

We have a very select amount of bacteria, or probiotics, on our gut mucosal lining, and all of them are like special SWAT TEAMs and assassins. I call these the Gut Guardians. They will selectively pick out pathogens, whether they're fungal, viral, bacterial or parasitic, and are amazing at killing them all off. Many of the strains of bacteria found in probiotics ward off things like giardia, *E. coli* and *Candida*.

So how does this relate to SIBO? If your small intestine has a very select amount of bacteria, when you start to exceed that count—as you do with SIBO—it's usually because you are missing these protective bacterial allies. After antibiotics, high stress or a high-sugar or a low-fiber diet, you'll be rather low on probiotics, especially ones from gooey starches and ancient grains. You might also be low on inulin-based fiber, which are found in almost 40,000 different plants like artichokes and asparagus.

SOIL-BASED PROBIOTICS IN HUMAN HISTORY

Probiotics are foods or supplements that contain "good" gut bacteria that help keep your gut healthy and balanced. Foods like yogurt can contain probiotics, and so can supplements. The most common of these supplemental probiotics are strains of Bifidobacteria and Lactobacillus.

Historically, one way we introduced probiotics into our system is through soil-based organisms. These organisms typically live in dirt, but can also exist in our digestive system.

What's so special about soil probiotics, specifically, and how are they important to our history? Our history as humans has always been intimately tied with dirt. In this dirt are probiotics, which protect all animals—insects, serpents, snakes and birds—because dirt is present everywhere. Back in the caveman days, humans didn't eat probiotics in a bottle—they just had dirt.

In today's world, we have to go backwards, look at how we used to integrate those probiotics and try to emulate it. One of the best ways to do this is by taking a soil-based organism probiotic.

"I was a wreck. Chronic fatigue was affecting every part of my life. I was so tired that I couldn't even read or go outside. I started using the Bifido Maximus and Prescript Assist probiotics daily from Dr.Grace, and my life changed in 8 weeks. After the probiotics, I have more energy and I can even tolerate more foods. After 6 weeks, I could go outside and walk again."

— DAVE A.

Something that is really neat about soil-based probiotics is that many come in spores, or hibernating life forms that can withstand all kinds of assault, like UV rays, high temperatures, low temperatures and even radiation. There are spores that were found 200 to 250 million years ago, and they're still viable. Because they last so long, scientists were are able to bloom them or grow them or open them up to look at their DNA.

Soil-based organism (SBO) probiotic spores self-populate in our gut, so once you start eating them regularly, they're constantly blooming for you. Even if you just maintain a dosing 1 or 2 times a week, they will continue to flourish. What's even better is that many of these strains of soil probiotics are found in naturally healthy microbiomes—they're supposed to be there to help protect your gut, so they are usually well-tolerated, even by people with severe SIBO.

At The Gut Institute, we carry a variety of soil-based probiotics, including the following:

— Equilibrium, 115-Strain Probiotic from General Biotics
— MegaSporebiotic, 5-Strain SBO Probiotic from Microbiome Labs
— Latero Flora, *Bacillus laterospòrus* BOD

Our online store iApothecary is our specialty boutique store for all things good for your gut microbiome! We carry several varieties of Soil-Based Organism (SBO) Probiotics. These require no refrigeration and mimic our intake of microbes from the environment. In Step 1 we talked about the importance of fermented foods. Several of these SBO strains are amplified in fermented legumes and beans such as Japanese fermented soybeans (known as natto) and ancestral Africa condiments and dishes (fermented beans). Our exposures to the environment and dirt are becoming less and less as we become more and more urbanized. Our microbiomes miss dirt. SBO Probiotics are key components found in healthy human and rural microbiome studies, but not in Westernized studies. It is naturally the best idea to gain these missing, vital connections to the outdoors through gardening, hiking, 'forest-bathing' and playing in the dirt with your children! Taking SBO Probiotics is also a fantastic way to gain these promises and payoffs from dirt!

— **Check them out here:**
https://thegutinstitute.com/equilibrium
https://thegutinstitute.com/megaspore
https://thegutinstitute.com/maximizekit

BENEFITS OF PROBIOTICS IN HUMAN CONTROLLED SIBO TRIALS

Some soil-based probiotic strains have been the focus of a few different studies that highlight their health benefits. One strain, Bacillus clausii, was tested in low doses in SIBO patients to determine how effective they were at reducing SIBO. One group of people took Bacillus clausii, and another group of people took antibiotics. In the end, the study showed that there was an equivalent number of SIBO reductions with probiotics compared to antibiotics. Practically half of the patients on probiotics were able to lower the markers of SIBO and reduce their gut distress symptoms. A meta-analysis with Lactobacilli and Bifidobacteria probiotics showed similar outcomes for SIBO treatment and pain relief. A pooled SIBO decontamination rate for 14 controlled trials was 62.8% observed in patients (range: 51.5% to 72.8%).

What studies like this one and many others show is that soil-based and traditional probiotics can be helpful in eradicating bad bacteria from the gut microbiome, easing symptoms of SIBO and working on maintaining gut flora balance. Since SIBO is in actuality also SIFO, fungal overgrowths, the hallmark features of probiotics for Step #3 is that they are also antifungal to potently and permanently ward off overgrowing yeasts and Candida.

Probiotics can also provide a bunch of other benefits because we are already supposed to have them in our gut. These bacteria work within our microbiomes to line the gut and protect it from pathogens and overgrowths. Probiotics are truly gut guardians. Studies also show they go and recruit higher concentrations of other gut guardians! Many also secrete 'sweet' food (exopolysaccharides) that other bacterial crew can consume between meals. The guardians are surprisingly altruistic.

Some other benefits include:

— Anti-inflammatories - These reduce joint and other chronic pain and free up energy to help you heal yourself.
— Increased nutrient absorption - You're able to get all the benefits of the healthy food you're eating.
— Immune system stimulation - Your immune system will be better prepared to fight off nasty germs and viruses.
— Antiparasitic chemicals - You will be less susceptible to the invasion of parasites that feed off your nutrient supply.
— Antipathogenic chemicals - These chemicals fight off disease-causing pathogens that may try to take over within your gut or come in from the outside world.

"I am about to start my second bottle of the Bifido Maximus Probiotic. I'm pretty much bedbound and have been ill for years. This is the first probiotic in 30 years of trying that I can really feel doing something. Thank you!"

— DR. BELINDA MARSH, DOCTOR AT NHS, FUNCTIONAL MEDICINE PRACTITIONER

THE MANY TYPES OF PROBIOTICS

The type of probiotics you take will be important if you have SIBO, because some types of bacteria may be more beneficial for your microbiome than others. There are lots of different strains of bacteria that might be found in probiotics: *Bacillus subtilis, Clostridium butyricum, Bifidobacteria longum, Lactobacillus plantarum and Bacillus clausii,* to name just a few. If you're taking a supplement, the specific bacteria included will be in the ingredients list.

Studies have also demonstrated the importance of choosing the correct type of probiotic. A group of scientists conducted a study a few years ago with children and babies who had a high risk of ADHD. They split the babies into two groups: one half got a probiotic containing *Lactobacillus rhamnosus* every day for 6 months starting at birth, and the other half got no probiotics. After administering probiotics for 6 months, they continued to monitor the children for 13 years and their stool compositions.

After the results were compiled and published, they found that 6 of the 35 children (17.1%) in the no-probiotic group were diagnosed with ADHD . In the other group that did receive probiotics, no children (0%)

developed ADHD. In other words 100% protection from ADHD. The results really generated a buzz.

What's even more fascinating about this study, though, is that it wasn't just the Lactobacillus rhamnosus probiotic that made the biggest difference. When they tested the stools of the children, they discovered 2 things. Stool composition as no different between the 2 groups except one thing. They found that the benefits of the probiotic were only found when *Bifidobacterium longum* was also present. There was an ADHD progression in children with no Bifidobacterium longum, whereas the children who had detectable levels of *Bifidobacterium longum*, as a result of the *Lactobacillus probiotic*, were shielded apparently from ADHD. The second finding was that the higher the *Bifidobacteria longum*, the higher the neuropsychological protection.

This shows us that there is a synergism that can happen between different types of probiotics. Many supplements will contain multiple strains that work together to provide you and your gut with the best possible health benefits.

I have a few probiotic supplement recommendations for people suffering from SIBO. Many of these products I have tried myself or am familiar with through The Gut Institute. The best way to take these probiotics is to rotate between different kinds every 3 to 5 days or every couple of weeks to get the numerous types of bacteria growing in your gut. Both ways develop diversity. I call it the Probiotic Parade.

The Gut Institute itself offers our signature Bifido Maximus Probiotic, which contains 7 strains that are all histamine-free and lactate-free strains. Our strains are powerful and compelling like those in mom's milk but gentle for everyone. Many of the strains also associated with supporting reduced *Candida*, parasites and oxalate degradation. For people who have different intolerances or inflammatory disorders, this is one of the best kinds of foundational probiotic strains. Bifido Maximus Probiotic is also special for building resilience. We challenge our clients to start eating gluten and dairy again after a few months to see what their intolerances are, and many people find that they can tolerate these substances without the wild and debilitating symptoms they had earlier. I am a fan of forever gluten-free and dairy-free lifestyles for those with high susceptible gut issues, but an occasional contamination should not make someone bed-bound or un-functional. I hope to rebuild resilience to the modern life after modern damages like antibiotics, pharmaceuticals and stress.

Another probiotic called Equilibrium is a great add-on soil-based probiotic. It has 115 strains, many of which are good *Eubacterium, Aeromonadaceae* and *Enterobacter* that we don't see as much in different probiotics. This one, in particular, seems to provide a great resilience for mood and helps improve happiness in my clients and observed in an in-house study.

Another favorite soil-based probiotic of mine is MegaSporebiotic, which contains 5 strains of Bacilli. The supplement contains 4 billion spores and is super powerful, helping to clarify the small intestines without causing many side effects. It's also super awesome for the skin, whether you suffer from psoriasis, acne or eczema.

Finally, Floraphage, another supplement, is not considered a probiotic. It's actually a prebiotic that causes bacteria to release nutrients that feed other beneficial gut flora. They're very targeted to enter toxic strains of *E. coli* in the gut. As these *E. coli* die off, they become food for *Bifidobacterium longum* and *Lactobacillus* and can amplify other probiotics for greater gut health.

If you want to give any of these supplements a try, they're all available at thegutinstitute.com.

"I am so grateful I found this probiotic. I have tried several in the past due to having Celiac disease and haven't noticed that they've helped. Recently I started a 6-week course of antibiotics and purchased this to take while going through treatment. I haven't experienced any of the gut discomfort that's usually associated with this antibiotic. It's nice to know that I'm getting the protection I need while going through treatment."

— MARCI

Building Up Your Probiotic Bacteria

There are a couple myths out there about probiotics, and one that I want to bust is the notion that probiotics are not necessary for SIBO treatment. This is simply not true. Even if you are in the "kill phase" of SIBO, where you're working to kill off the excess bacteria in your gut, probiotics can be a big help. While this may seem counterintuitive—to add bacteria to the gut while you're trying to decrease the bacterial overgrowth—taking the right kind of probiotics can help.

The whole reason people develop SIBO is because of our

modern world filled with antibiotics and lacking those soil-based organisms we used to get from the dirt. Antibiotics wipe out the probiotics we need as allies to protect our gut mucosal lining. Taking probiotics can help re-introduce those early on.

Whether someone is really reactive to a specific probiotic will really depend on how severe their SIBO is. Around 10% or higher percentage of all SIBO cases involve overgrowth of Lactobacilli, so those people may not be able to tolerate our Bifido Maximus Probiotic foundational probiotic or others containing Lactobacilli. Too much of a good thing occurs once the true guardians are gone. The Lactobacilli in the overgrowth may produce excessive lactate are usually the bad kind that eat sugar and carbs rather than fiber. Bifido Maximus is lactate-free strains and often can be tolerated at very tiny amounts without histamine reactions and gradually increased.

The same kind of thing might occur with Bifidobacteria — severe dysbiosis in the gut might result in a Bifido intolerance. In cases like these, some caution will need to be exercised. Trying a probiotic is sort of a litmus test to see what you can tolerate and what you can't.

When you start taking probiotics, it's good to layer them on one by one. Start with a foundational probiotic, especially if you are missing a lot of Bifidobacteria and Lactobacilli in your microbiome. If you have more severe SIBO, look for a soil-based probiotic that won't irritate the existing bacterial overgrowth.

Then, depending on your tolerance, you can start to layer on other probiotics based on what your gut's needs are. In time, you should begin to experience fewer symptoms of SIBO and be that much closer to maintaining a healthy microbiome.

Don't forget to take the free 7-day companion course video lessons and check out the extra information at HealSIBO.com.

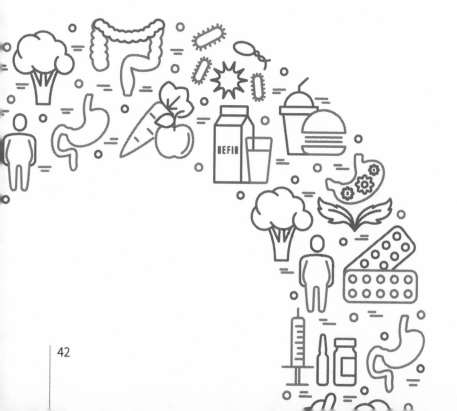

CHAPTER 4

Fueling Your Bacteria with Bionic Fiber

Small intestinal bacterial overgrowth, or SIBO, affects a growing number of people each day. The rise in SIBO is largely due to the use of antibiotics, which wipe out good and bad gut flora, as do periods of high stress or poor diet. While SIBO can cause a variety of unpleasant symptoms, you may be surprised to discover that it also plays a large role in sudden weight gain. Later, we'll discuss why this happens, and I'll give you a tip to reverse it.

REFLECTING ON OUR PREVIOUS STEPS TOWARD HEALTH

We've reached Step 4 of my 7-step process for reducing or overcoming SIBO. By now, we've started to introduce small amounts of gut-friendly foods like fermented products and ancient grains and starches into our diets. Step 3 took it a step further to begin growing colonies of healthy gut bacteria using soil-based probiotics.

This 7-step method aims to recolonize and reset the natural rhythms of your body. Each step may not cure your SIBO completely, but together, they will help make your gut so much stronger and more robust. A healthy gut microbiome creates a type of armor for your health so that you can amp up to an even higher level.

If you've been experiencing discomfort with the last few steps, continue to take it slow and work up to larger amounts. When you find a point where you feel comfortable and your gut is able to tolerate the new levels of healthy bacteria you're introducing, you're ready for Step 4, where you'll really start to fuel these good bacteria so they work to make you healthy.

HOW SIBO CAN AFFECT YOUR WEIGHT

One of the symptoms that Step 4, in particular, can help reduce is sudden fat gain brought about by SIBO. I've struggled with SIBO numerous times throughout my life. In my teens and 20s, I was suffering from low energy, bloating and weight gain with no relief.

Over time, as I aged, I got healthier and did a lot of things that actually ramped up my health. I lost 50 pounds, gained 10 to 20 pounds of muscle mass and was stronger and more defined than I had ever been. I didn't know it at the time, but the things I was doing were helping my gut reset and find balance.

The reason I experienced this weight gain and bloating was due to SIBO, SIFO and the bad flora that came along with it. When you have overgrowths, the bad gut flora that eat sugar and simple carbs take over. If you don't have good bacteria to push these bad guys out, they keep growing, leading to symptoms like weight gain, the inability to gain muscle mass, bloating and fatigue. This can eventually lead to a number of conditions including autoimmunity, mood and hormone disorders, and cancer.

This happens because of increased inflammation and toxic parasitic microbes that begin to enter the bloodstream. Toxic fungi will also grow in abundance and result in a cascade of problems. These bad flora and their bad chemicals and cell components raise blood sugars, cause insulin resistance, intestinal permeability ('leaky gut'), and begin to accumulate fat and even affect your liver.

However, all of these problems are reversible if we take control of our gut microbiomes, introduce new, good bacteria and fuel them with super-foods. So what exactly is this super fuel for good bacteria? What do the bacteria really want so they can produce the wonderful vitamins and chemicals that help our bodies? The answer is simple: fiber.

STEP 4 TO OVERCOMING SIBO

Eating Prebiotic Fiber

One of the best things to eat that can help you fuel your gut bacteria is fiber. We touched on this during Step 2 with ancient grains. Cooked ancient grains contain a compound called resistant starch (RS3), which is a type of prebiotic fiber that your gut flora loves.

When you eat these types of fiber, it ferments in the digestive system, feeding bacteria that produce short-chain fatty acids. These acids then fuel your mucosal lining bacteria, which fortify the gut. Feeding these types of bacteria will force the bad flora out, making your gut microbiome healthy and balanced once again.

Well, resistant starch is not the only kind of prebiotic fiber. In fact, many soluble fibers (fibers that can dissolve in water) are able to ferment in your colon, as well, providing nourishment for the flora in your mucosal lining. For example, inulin and oligosaccharides, composed of chains of simple sugars, are prebiotics that are found naturally in tons of plants. Oligosaccharides are also found in the bran and germination areas of grains, seeds, beans, tubers, as well as cactus. Cooked, gooey versions are the best for the bacteria! They mimic mucus in our intestines. Mother Nature uses oligosaccharides to protect the precious legacy of her plants from drying out and weather extremes studies show. What is good for plants is good for our us, just like other plant substances like plant antioxidants and phytosterols.

"I spent 2 years of my life trying to figure out why I struggled to digest many common foods. Despite trying many different diets (Paleo, GAPS, keto, etc.) and cooking everything myself, I still experienced IBS symptoms on a daily basis. It wasn't until I came across Dr. Grace's work that I turned the corner. Understanding the microbiome was my missing link to improved gut health, and Dr. Grace is the most knowledgeable expert with the most effective strategies on the topic that I encountered. Specifically, taking a soil-based probiotic (Prescript Assist), while adding cooked resistant starches and bionic fiber resulted in less stomach discomfort, improved bowel movements and, most importantly, the ability to reintroduce foods I wasn't able to digest prior. It's a great feeling to be able to sit down and share a meal with friends and family again.
Thanks, Dr. Grace!"

— J.W.

CREATING YOUR OWN 'BIONIC FIBER'

To implement more of these awesome prebiotic fibers into your diet, try "bionic fiber." This is something I concocted, and it's a great way to give your gut flora all the super fuels it needs to do everything it possibly can for you. As a mixture of powdered fibers, bionic fiber can nourish your good bacteria and even help resurrect good flora that were low in numbers before.

There are a lot of different powdered fibers to choose from, and you can mix and match to create your own unique blend of prebiotics. Aim for a diverse set of fibers for the best results.

Here are a few of my personal favorites:

— Organic psyllium husk
— Inulin and FOS (fructo-oligosaccharides)
— Glucomannan
— MegaPrebiotic from Microbiome Laboratory
— MetaFiber from Metagenics
— PaleoFiber Berry from Designs For Health
— Raw Reserve Berry Extracts

Psyllium comes from the seed husks of a hearty plant (a weed in fact) called Plantago ovata. Two fantastic facts about this fiber is that it is (1) one of the few that contains both soluble and insoluble fiber, so it has multiple ways to nourish the microbiome. (2) Secondly, psyllium is one of the few prebiotics shown to bind toxins, lower body fat, control blood sugars, improves insulin sensitivity and lowers small, dense LDL-cholesterol ('bad') in human trials.

Inulin powder is one of my favorites because it tastes a little sweet and it's super gooey. The gooey texture is what our gut flora love, because the mucus that line our GI tract from tongue-to-tail is where the protective gut flora live is also gooey and contain special sugar, fucose. Additionally, inulin has been shown in human trials to improve inflammation patterns, benefit digestive disorders and proliferate all of our bacterial guardians. Inulin contains some FOS, short for fructo-oligosaccharides. FOS is powerful. FOS can also be cooked down or extracted from rich sources such as yacon root, cacti and fruits.

Glucomannan is from a root called Konjac, which is often eaten in Asia. It's a super gooey, starchy root that gets even gooier when cooked. This has prebiotic fiber that has been shown to reduce body fat and the risk for diabetes and cancer. However, glucomannan expands a lot and needs to be accompanied by a lot of water. Many people can only handle a very small amount of glucomannan in the beginning because it really can swell up. We use only a tiny amount in bionic fiber. A little goes a long way.

Some products like MegaPrebiotic, MetaFiber and PaleoFiber have a blend of diverse soluble fibers. If you're mixing fibers yourself, though, and don't like the flavor, you can add something like green or red berry powder. One of my favorites is called Raw Reserve, which comes in different flavors. It's actually a synbiotic, because it contains both prebiotics and probiotics.

If you don't want to purchase things like powdered fibers, it's not a problem! You can continue to add cooked starches and fibrous vegetables into your diet. If you're able to tolerate small amounts, try adding a little more and see how your gut reacts.

"Dr. Grace's fiber combo fit right in with my blood sugar regulation protocol and cured the problem. Fiber certainly helps shed weight, too, and makes it easier to keep weight off. I am no longer a snacker, which was the reason for my weight gain. Your fibers are a saving grace (pun intended) when it comes to fasting, and fasting is a wonderful tool to get the fat carved off quickly. My stomach is flatter now than it has been in years without me going gaunt all over."

— J.P.

Let Fiber Do the Work For You

A lot of guts love bionic fiber to feed them and promote gut lining protection. With this kind of super fuel, your microbiome will become even more balanced and you should be able to tolerate additional kinds of foods thanks to a well-functioning gut.

When you're working on adding bionic fiber, consider taking a small amount of powdered fiber, one type at a time, and mix it with water every other day. Gradually, you can begin to increase the amount of fiber you add, but it's a good idea to start slow to test your tolerance.

Within a few weeks, you should be able to notice a difference in the way your gut reacts to foods, as well as changes in your SIBO symptoms. Your tummy may be flatter, and you might start to feel better and much more energetic. Symptom reduction will start to link up together because your microbiome is getting happier and happier, and that's our whole goal. If your microbiome is happy, you're going to be happy.

Don't forget to take the free 7-day companion course video lessons and check out the extra information at HealSIBO.com.

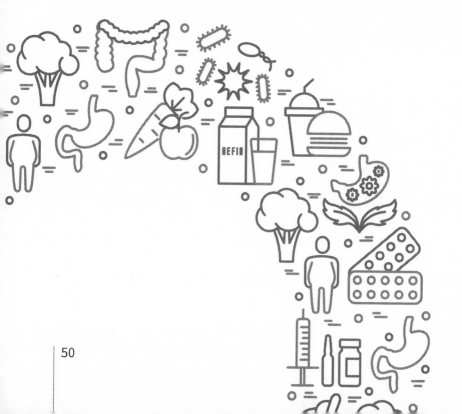

CHAPTER 5

Stepping Your Way to a Healthier Gut

SIBO, or small intestinal bacterial overgrowth, can cause a wide range of symptoms in patients. This overgrowth of bad bacteria in the gut can lead to problems like irritable bowel syndrome, stomach cramps and diarrhea, as well as release toxic chemicals that affect the way your entire body functions.

These days, not only are we "free" of all the good gut flora, but we're also overrun with bad, pathogenic flora. We have firewalls in our gut that protect from invaders getting in, but if those are down—if our good gut flora is gone—anything you might encounter can invade and colonize your body, making things go awry.

Previously, we've discussed steps you can take to minimize the effects and actually reverse SIBO by introducing and feeding our natural probiotics and protective allies in the gut mucosal lining. Through the introduction of helpful acids, probiotics and super fuel prebiotics, you will have set the stage for your gut to rebalance itself.

This next step can take your gut microbiome balance to the next level and help you overcome challenges with both SIBO and painful cramping in the gut.

THE SCIENCE OF MITOCHONDRIA AND YOUR MICROBIOME

Step 5 in my 7-step process is something that will not only benefit your gut flora and balance your microbiome, but will also benefit your mitochondria. As you may remember from school, the mitochondria are the "powerhouse" of your cells. You may not realize this, but they're nearly identical to bacteria found in your gut microbiome.

Anything that is bad for your muscles and mitochondria is also quite bad for your microbiome. This connection may not seem obvious, but our mitochondria actually used to be bacteria.

During endocytosis (the process cells use to engulf matter and transport it), our cells actually took over one of the smallest intracellular bacterium, known as rickettsiae, and used this bacterium as a nuclear powerhouse to make energy. Rickettsiae became this factory that can burn fat and make a lot of ATP, or energy, for us. This is the simplest, most primitive alchemy that happens at the cellular level.

In terms of pharmaceuticals, any drugs that are toxic to mitochondria are also going to be toxic for your microbiome. There are a whole host of these kinds of drugs, such as statin drugs used to lower cholesterol and chemotherapy agents to kill cancer cells, as well as antibiotics. We know antibiotics kill bacteria, but it turns out that they also have side effects that make them super toxic for your mitochondria.

Muscles have are densely populated with mitochondria for energy demands. This leads us to the analogy that if we can prime our muscles and mitochondria and make them happy, our microbiome will be happy, too. This can result in great gut changes and a reduction of SIBO.

Exercise Regularly

One way we can make both of these systems happy is through exercise. Exercise is not just essential for whole-body health—it is one of the most important things you can do for your gut health, since the kind of exercise that ramps up your mitochondria also ramps up your microbiome.

Exercise has been linked to increases in good bacteria in the gut, which we already know fortify the mucosal lining and prevent pathogens from taking over. Studies have shown that people who routinely exercise have much greater diversity in their gut flora and much more protective bacteria than people who don't exercise much or at all.

Exercise also has another benefit related to SIBO, which is to improve the ways our gut moves food through and out of our body.

HOW YOUR GUT MOVES ITS CONTENTS

There are two main ways that food and mucus move through the small intestine that might be affected by SIBO. One way is through peristalsis, or involuntary waves and contractions that push the contents of the intestine forward.

The peristalsis is a weak, wiggly kind of movement related to the smooth muscle lining your intestinal tract. Anything that is autonomic, or that we're not really thinking about, moves your smooth muscle. Our bodies can do these types of movements even if we're not awake, so it doesn't require any conscious thought at all.

The other way gut contents move is through the MMC, which stands for the migrating motor complex. The third wave of MMC is a different kind of contraction than the peristalsis, transmitted through neurologic electrical signals from the brain. MMC is pretty powerful and actually shuttles all the bacteria along the GI tract forward so it doesn't retrograde, or go backwards into your small intestine or stomach. I like to think of these contraction waves as "housekeeping" waves because they help to clean out the food and bad bacteria from the gut, which can benefit people with SIBO.

The MMC usually has rhythmic contractions that are painless. People normally don't even notice it. However, in more severe conditions like IBS, SIBO or other bowel inflammation, these contractions may be disrupted, and that can lead to cramping or uncomfortable feelings.

Take The 10,000 Steps A Day Challenge

For Step 5 on your way to overcoming SIBO, I challenge you to work up to taking 10,000 steps a day. This is about 5 miles, but you can obviously split up the time it takes to reach this goal throughout the day. Take multiple 10- or 15-minute walks, or do larger stints to reach the big goal.

What I love about 10,000 steps is that it's very close to what our ancestors probably did in their day. They had plenty of rest time, as well, which we may get if we're lucky. But we might not always be getting the workout, the exercise that moves and strengthens our microbiome and our mitochondria.

If you are someone who is bed-bound or suffers from chronic fatigue, this goal will take some time to meet, and that's okay. If you cannot move much, start your goal low and go slow. For your particular mitochondria and your microbiome, even doing 10 steps a day can make a massive improvement toward overcoming SIBO.

Life is full of different opportunities to meet this challenge and do the steps every day. Here are some ideas to help you reach the goal:

— Park your car a little further away and walk to your destination

— Take a short, 10-minute walk every hour

— Take the stairs in a high-rise building instead of the elevator

— Bring music with you on walks or to the gym to make it more fun

Standing while at work instead of sitting can sometimes help, too, but it is a little static. The movements where you're using your big muscles and pumping blood are what your mitochondria and microbiome want. Our mitochondria love oxygen. That's how they burn fat for us, through aerobic metabolic activity.

Your colon only houses anaerobic gut flora, or bacteria that don't like oxygen. However, your small intestine has more oxygen-using bacteria, which is another way exercise can help regulate your gut. Oxygen is antimicrobial and antifungal—it flushes out all tissues and can help kill pathogens.

If you're like me, you like to track things. I love to use my smartphone to track my steps. Other people have a Fitbit or Apple Watch. There are so many different, amazing apps to help you track whether or not you're getting in 10,000 steps a day.

Ultimately, you'll just need to find out what works for you. It can also help to find a good reward for yourself for getting up to that 10,000 steps goal—just make sure it's not a food reward.

If you are experiencing SIBO with side effects like chronic fatigue, brain fog or fat burning issues, exercise can help right it with the help of probiotics. Using this step in conjunction with all the previous steps, you should start to see small changes in your gut that help you look better and feel better.

Don't forget to take the free 7-day companion course video lessons and check out the extra information at HealSIBO.com.

CHAPTER 6

Preventing Leaky Gut By Avoiding Toxic Foods

People who suffer from small intestinal bacterial overgrowth (SIBO) and small intestinal fungal overgrowth (SIFO) often find that their bodies react negatively to particular foods. You may say you are "sensitive" to a food, like gluten, eggs or dairy. This is why many restricted food diets like the paleo diet help people regulate their painful digestive tract symptoms.

What a lot of people don't realize is that these foods might be allergens for your body, meaning they provoke an allergic reaction in the immune system. Additionally, eating these allergenic foods doesn't always result in an upset stomach or diarrhea. It can also trigger more "silent" symptoms, like brain fog, chronic fatigue, bad moods and weight gain, that you might not inherently link to your diet.

But what causes these sensitivities? Typically, an imbalance in your gut microbiome is to blame. If you have all the healthy probiotics and a strong gut mucosal lining, you should be able to eat many of these foods without symptoms. If you suffer from SIBO, though, you'll need to do some work to get there.

Steps 1 through 5 of my 7-step process for overcoming SIBO are working to prime your gut with healthy bacteria and nourishment to strengthen and balance out the gut flora. You might still need some time to really see results. Some people start to see symptoms fading away in as little as a week, but others with more severe cases will take longer.

Many of these steps will need to happen simultaneously to help the healthy bacteria really "anchor" in your intestines. Keep working on eating fermented foods, ancient grains, probiotics and fiber while exercising to continue in your path to a healthy gut.

Rather than adding something to your daily routine, Step 6 in the process actually has to do with removing things. Specifically, I'm going to be talking about removing toxic foods from your diet. Some of these might actually shock you, but eliminating them might put you on the path to helping you feel better.

"I'm a 45-year-old male. For years I've had difficulty gaining muscle mass and lowering HDL cholesterol. I was stuck, I was doing ketosis and successfully went from 230 to 200 lbs, which had worked for me previously, but I stopped losing weight and I felt horrible. Two months ago, I changed my diet after reading about bionic fiber and added in more protein, fruits and vegetables, lowered saturated fat and added in the Bionic Fiber protocol and the ultra potent Bifido Maximus Probiotic. I used two bottles of Bifido Maximus and feel better than ever. My liver test ALT went from 60

to 17 in two months and I went from 200 lbs to 180. I am
so pleased with my new body and lifestyle."

— **BRUCE M., BAY AREA, CALIFORNIA**

Types of Toxic Foods for the Body

Two of the worst offenders in your gut are allergens and chemicals that shouldn't be eaten in the first place. These types of foods might be okay for the average person every once in a while, but most of us eat these foods too often, which can lead to the formation of gut dysbiosis, SIBO, SIFO and leaky gut syndrome.

WHAT IS LEAKY GUT?

Leaky gut happens when the lining of the small intestine becomes damaged, allowing undigested food, toxic chemicals and bacteria to enter the bloodstream. The tight junctions in your gut act like gateways and control what passes through this lining, but when you have leaky gut, they aren't able to work properly.

It only takes a small problem with leaky gut to develop more major health issues. The things that don't belong in the bloodstream trigger the immune system, and your body does what it's supposed to do: it tries to launch attacks against them. This results in inflammation, which can cause even worse leaky gut, leading to a vicious cycle in the body.

Over time, this takes a big toll on your health. If your body is spending so much energy and time fighting against foreign objects in the bloodstream, that means less energy is spent on processing nutrients and healing your body.

Leaky gut and food allergies or toxic foods are often correlated because the allergens can cause inflammation in your gut, damaging that intestinal lining. However, this doesn't happen as much when you have the good bacteria in your gut to help break down these substances and quell inflammation before it causes problems.

ALLERGENIC FOODS

When you think of the word "allergy," you might immediately picture someone reacting to an allergy through anaphylaxis, which can cause difficulty breathing and be life-threatening. However, an "allergy" indicates an abnormal reaction from our immune system to an otherwise-harmless substance.

When someone initially comes into contact with allergens like nuts or eggs, a white blood cell in the body called the B-lymphocyte makes antibodies, which the body can retain in its memory. Severe allergies occur when the body produces immunoglobulin E (IgE) and tags the particular food.

When I refer to food allergens here, I mean those that result in a change in immunoglobulin G, or IgG (a type of antibody produced by the B-lymphocyte). These IgGs indicate a sensitivity or intolerance from the body when they are high, which is something you can have tested with an IgG food panel. We can reverse these types of intolerances by taking care of the gut.

Apart from food allergens that might be super toxic to you, if you look at your IgG food panel, the top three reactants are the most lethal foods for your gut and can kill the gut lining. Fortunately, a prevalence of probiotics and a healthy gut can fix this intolerance, allowing you to eat some of these allergenic foods again.

GMO FOODS

The second group of foods that is really toxic for the gut is the GMO foods, or genetically-modified organisms. GMO foods have been altered to ward off diseases and pests and are extremely common in today's world. Many grains, like wheat, as well as vegetable and seed oils, are genetically modified and can be harmful to your gut microbiome.

Many crops have death genes and they are not great for us to eat, nor is it great for any of our gut flora to transform and have those genes put into them. A lot of crops that are genetically altered also spew out horrible chemicals and pesticides, which are linked to multiple chronic conditions like autoimmune diseases and cancer. Pesticides are essentially antibiotics for plants and keep pests away, but not all "pests" are really pests. When these chemicals enter the body, they can kill off the good bacteria in your gut, leaving the bad kinds of bacteria and yeast behind.

These chemicals also don't go away easily. Some studies have shown that these pesticides show up in the people who eat them. One study in particular indicated detectable rates of pesticides inside pregnant moms and their fetuses.

Unfortunately, GMOs are a reality in our world, so how do we deal with them? Probiotics are shown to break down pesticides. Another, better option is to eat organic or home-grown crops that do not have these pesticides in them. For ultimate health, try to eliminate these types of foods entirely.

Eliminate Toxic Foods

This may be tough to swallow—no pun intended—but you may actually be reacting to the foods you love to consume every day. For Step 6 in this process to help you overcome SIBO, you're going to want to take action against the foods that may be causing your body harm by removing them from your diet.

It's very important to know what kinds of specific foods your body reacts to. You can identify these foods through an IgG food panel test like we offer at The Gut Institute, or you can do elimination tests on your own at home to help you figure out what foods you're sensitive to.

So, what happens when you remove these foods from your diet? Elimination of toxic foods (paired with ingestion of probiotics!) will help your body stop producing IgG antibodies for a specific allergen. Sometimes, it takes extra work to dissolve the immune complexes, which retain the memory. Eventually, these complexes get broken down and your body absorbs them. Not eating these allergenic foods helps you produce more energy, since your body won't be fighting off the allergen.

Ultimately, your body is going to be able to heal a lot faster. Removing the sources of inflammation and havoc in your gut will allow the probiotics and healthy bacteria to thrive and repair your microbiome. Then, when your gut is healed again thanks to the good bacteria, you should be able to slowly reintroduce these foods back into your diet without experiencing those intolerances.

THE TASK: PICK ONE TOXIC FOOD AND REMOVE IT

Your challenge for this step is this: consider choosing 1 of these toxic gut foods and eliminate it from your diet for just 4 weeks.

To help you start, here are 3 of the most toxic gut foods:

— Gluten (most types of bread, pasta, cookies, cake, beer and deep fried foods)

— GMO corn (high fructose corn syrup, which is used to sweeten a lot of foods)

— Dairy (cheese, milk and butter)

I'd recommend that almost anybody remove 1 of these foods for at least the first month of their gut healing, because they are so commonly toxic to people. If you want to go the extra mile, consider eliminating all 3 of these foods for the month.

If you want to go super hardcore on this step, you can consider other types of foods that might be causing your gut harm, such as non-organic meat. Try switching to pasture-raised meat instead. Also, you might want to replace any of your vegetable and seed oils. Any of these hydrogenated fats are toxic to your gut flora. Instead, try using extra virgin olive oil, pork fat, lard or chicken fat.

Finally, if you want to be extremely hardcore with this step, remove nuts and eggs from your diet for a month. So many people are allergic or have mild sensitivities to these foods and don't even realize it, but eat them so often. This usually results in seemingly-unrelated symptoms and low energy that can be fixed when they are not eaten anymore.

"Around 3 years ago, I was diagnosed with diverticulitis. At least 4 episodes happened where I was in excruciating pain in my stomach and abdomen. I would get flu-like symptoms. I'd get a fever and could hardly move. The last episode I had was in October. I was actually at Disneyland and I started getting horrible pain in my left side. Then I had a fever and ended up in the hospital for 5 days. I had an abscess. After that they told me they wanted to do surgery. I talked to my chiropractor, Dr. Ron. He recommended that I talk to Dr. Grace Liu. Her gut class program helped me so I didn't have to have surgery.

Yes, I did the Organic Acid Test (OAT) and blood IgG test to find out what I'm probably allergic to and other things that were going on in the gut that you don't get at the conventional doctor. They came back that I was allergic to gluten and dairy, and there were some other things that were high. Dr. Liu had put me on a protocol regimen of different supplements, and I cut out the gluten, the dairy and a lot of sugar. I also cut down my caffeine intake.

I lost 30 pounds in less than 2 months.

She wanted me to try walking. I have so much more energy. I used to have achy muscles and joints all the time. I was telling my husband last night that I went out and pulled weeds. Usually I would go into this real pain for almost a week. I'm recovering faster without pain. One of the first times when I felt all this energy, I felt like I was this crazy woman. I was going through the house doing all this stuff. I told my husband, 'This is what I would be like if I was normal.'

Thank you for all that you do."

— **CARRIE ZIMMER, WALNUT CREEK, CA**

BENEFITS OF REMOVING TOXIC FOODS FROM YOUR DIET

The dangers of eating GMO foods loaded with pesticides or allergenic foods that cause inflammation in your gut are clear. These types of foods will harm your gut mucosal lining, allowing bacteria and viruses into the bloodstream, and harm the gut flora themselves. All of these problems can result in a myriad of health effects you might feel for years.

Besides the tightening of your gut lining and a more healthy microbiome, stopping leaky gut, eliminating these toxic foods can provide plenty of additional health benefits:

- Increased energy and endurance
- Increased carbohydrate tolerance
- Calmer and happier moods
- Reduced agitation
- Reduced anxiety
- Improved sleeping
- Weight loss
- Decreased acne and wrinkles

Reintroducing Foods

Start Step 6 by removing 1 of these toxic foods, or more if you're feeling ambitious. You might start to feel better right away, within a week. Some people will take longer, but don't give up. Keep avoiding these toxic foods and continue eating the helpful foods from Steps 1 through 5, unless they are a source of your sensitivity (such as histamine in fermented foods).

The process will eventually seal the gateways in your gut that cause leaky gut and other health problems due to inflammation. After 4 to 6 weeks, you can start to slowly reintroduce these types of foods into your diet and see how your body reacts. If you eliminated multiple foods, add 1 food back in per week so you can adequately monitor your reactions.

Over time, when the probiotics are firmly anchored in place in your gut and the microbiome has rebalanced after SIBO, you should have very little issue eating these types of foods again. You can eventually be able to enjoy the foods you love without the negative consequences.

Don't forget to take the free 7-day companion course video lessons and check out the extra information at HealSIBO.com.

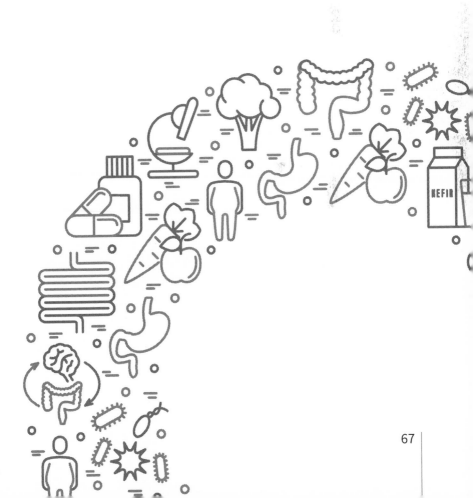

CHAPTER 7

Solidifying a Healthy Gut By Reducing Stress

Hippocrates once said, "All disease begins in the gut." And he was right—your digestive system is inherently linked to the health of your entire body. After all, over 70% of your immune system comes from the gut. Digestion and the absorption of nutrients that help your body run and make energy happen there, too. If you really think about it, it makes tons of sense that an unhealthy gut could lead to problems throughout the entire body—not just stomach cramps, constipation and bloating.

From heavy doses of antibiotics and medical practices, to unbalanced health and immune systems, to modern, sterile lifestyles, to a naturally-occuring lack of probiotics, there are a lot of ways that we can develop SIBO and its partner in crime, SIFO (small intestinal fungal overgrowth).

Despite his anatomical accuracy, though, I disagree somewhat with Hippocrates. I would say it is actually longevity that begins in the gut. SIBO is not a permanent condition. We can change this all around and mimic our ancestral roots to rebalance our gut microbiomes. We are capable of fixing these problems to promote lifelong health.

ADDING UP ALL THE STEPS TOWARD GUT HEALTH

This 7-step process for overcoming SIBO is a good one to follow to attempt to regulate your gut flora and get them back on track. If you've been following along for all the steps and have begun incorporating them into your everyday routine, you might already be seeing some changes, and that's great!

If you haven't seen much progress yet, don't worry. Some people have more severe cases than others and require a bit more attention. Assessing your progress and the ways your body has reacted to each step is a good litmus test for where your gut is right now and where it can be in the future.

In Step 1, we started out by adding fermented foods to your diet. These foods introduce natural acids, enzymes and some healthy gut bacteria to get the process of recolonizing your gut started.

Then, in Step 2, we moved on to ancient grains, which contain resistant starch that superfuels the bacteria in your gut mucosal lining.

In Step 3, you added soil-based probiotics to your regimen. These probiotics introduce the most natural, ancient gut bacteria that we are likely missing today due to antibiotics and our ultra-clean lifestyles.

Step 4 had you begin taking "bionic fiber," your own personal mix of prebiotic fiber, to feed your probiotics and get them ready to defend your colon.

Step 5 got you up and moving as you worked up to taking 10,000 steps a day. All this exercise can reduce inflammation in the gut and help resurrect nearly-gone probiotics.

Finally, in Step 6, I asked you to consider removing 1 or more toxic foods from your diet for a month to help fix leaky gut and retrain your immune system to accept what used to be your food sensitivities.

Now, we're talking about Step 7, the final step to overcoming SIBO. Up until now, each step has been about adding to or removing something from your routine. You've been taking lots of action. But it's not just what you eat and what you do that impacts your gut health. Surprisingly, it's also about your mindset.

STEP 7 TO OVERCOMING SIBO

Establish a Mind-Gut Connection

The seventh and final step in this process has to do with the connection between your mind and your gut microbiome. We are aware that SIBO can affect your mood, causing anxiety, depression, brain fog and mood swings, but it can also go the other way around. Stress plays a major role in the health of your gut flora.

The adrenal glands in your body produce a few different hormones when you are stressed. When you have high levels of epinephrine, adrenaline, norepinephrine and cortisol, you are at a higher risk of developing leaky gut and other gut-related problems.

Modern medicine uses a lot of hormonal steroids as treatment, which can be awesome, but they also can instantly damage your gut, causing leaky gut and ulcers. There is no organ system that is going to be free from cortisol damage, and it's the same way with the gut.

In contrast, 80% of your serotonin, the happy transmitter, comes from your gut as a product of good probiotics. Melatonin, the hormone helpful for sleep, is also made from serotonin. Serotonin, dopamine and adrenaline levels can all be affected if you lack the healthy bacteria in your gut to produce them, which results in a lot of bodily dysfunction. Males can experience low testosterone counts, while women may experience menstrual irregularity, and even fertility can be affected.

Fortunately, you can help reverse these problems by working to manage your stress and recolonize your healthy gut flora.

TYPES OF STRESSES

Stress isn't just caused by running late for work or having monetary or personal troubles. There are tons of types of stresses that your body will endure throughout your lifetime, prompting the production of stress hormones like cortisol.

One type of stress is obvious: the mental and physical stressors that are associated with everyday life or trauma. Getting into a car accident, losing your job or dealing with a painful breakup forces your adrenal glands to kick into overdrive. Chronic pain can also be extremely stressful. Some of this pain may even be caused by SIBO, which is all the more reason to work to eliminate it.

Additionally, eating foods that are bad for you can put stress on the body. Foods that we talked about for Step 6—like GMO foods or allergenic foods—can mess with your body, especially if they are gluten, dairy, eggs or GMO corn.

Any pathogenic organism or virus that sneaks into your body is also stressful. To truly combat these, you need a solid foundation of probiotics, which actually lowers when your stress is too high.

Plain and simple, the effects of stress are terrible for your gut microbiome and your body. It can break your gut and abruptly change your gut flora to a more pathogenic pattern.

Finding Ways to Regulate Stress

If stress is a one-way-ticket to an unhealthy gut microbiome, then you need to have a plan in place to manage it when it inevitably comes along. There are lots of ways we can do this, and they will largely vary by the individual, but I have a few really effective suggestions.

YOGA

First, you should try yoga. Yoga has been practiced for millennia—there are so many cultures that engage in all different kinds of yoga. The most ancient styles, in particular, are so deeply healing. When you start, you might want to try a few different types to find the right one for you.

I love yoga and have been doing it on and off for around 15 years. What I've noticed throughout the years is that when I'm off yoga, my health and my gut start to tank rapidly. If I am able to do it regularly, even just one or two times a week, then my gut and body feel pretty good. There are lots of benefits to yoga that many other people, in addition to myself, have experienced. It is one of the best tools I have found for getting the sympathetic nervous system and sympathetic drive to calm down and rest.

However, I recommend that you avoid certain types of exercise during periods of adrenal stress because they could have negative effects. One of these is Bikram yoga, which can get very hot. Another is cold thermogenesis, or dipping yourself in ice water. Any type of extreme or endurance exercise is probably not going to help regulate your hormones. Instead, it will just make them worse.

ADAPTOGENS

Another method that is great for your hormones and is known to lower stress is taking adaptogens. These are chemical signals in plants that you can take as botanical extracts. Adaptogens are known to help buffer stress and provide energy and mental clarity to people.

Many of these botanicals are antioxidants for plants and can even increase their antioxidant properties if the plant is under extreme stress. Our good gut flora also love antioxidants. They flourish because it's like a super food for them.

There are tons of different types of adaptogens. Not all of them will work for everyone, so you might need to try a few to find the right fit—just like with yoga. A few options include:

— Ashwagandha

— Rhodiola

— Ginseng

— Cordyceps

— Reishi

At the Gut Institute, we recommend that all our clients have a source of adaptogens to help fight off the effects of chronic stress. Using natural botanicals like the ones listed above are great—you can cook with them or add them to smoothies.

Another product we love is called NanoMojo. This is an amazing adaptogen that has over 20 botanicals mixed in at tiny doses. Our clients have loved it in the past, and almost all of them have reported amazing benefits from it. It can help provide more energy and endurance, normalize your menstrual cycle, help you lose weight and help you relax.

Check out our iApothecary products for your Mind-Gut Axis!

https://thegutinstitute.com/nanomojo
https://thegutinstitute.com/dragonmojo
https://thegutinstitute.com/perfectpoop [complimentary probiotic]
https://thegutinstitute.com/mycotaki

STRESS LESS ABOUT YOUR BODY AND YOUR GUT

People with SIBO know that the condition can be stressful. The varying symptoms such as brain fog, constipation, diarrhea or chronic pain can seriously drive you nuts. All this stress just leads to more problems in the gut, leading to more stress… and the cycle continues.

By finding ways to manage your stress—and by extension, your hormones and adrenal glands—you'll be that much closer to eliminating your problems with SIBO.

Continue to work on all the steps in this process by implementing good, gut-friendly foods, probiotics and exercise to benefit your microbiome. You may be just around the corner from a drastic change in your health!

The Gut Institute Can Help

Unfortunately, my 7-step process for overcoming SIBO isn't going to work for everyone. You may have a very severe case, be unsure of how to begin or just not have access to products you need to rebuild your microbiome. Or, the process is working, but you're looking for a way to cement your progress permanently and to built gut resilience. Everyone is different and has different needs in their battle with SIBO. Regardless of these needs, I may have a solution for you.

The Gut Institute, a platform for education and research about the gut microbiome and how it relates to longevity, offers classes and other resources to help put you on the path to better health. Our goal isn't just about getting you to look and feel good—it's about being productive, following your passions, building better relationships and having a better quality of life across the board. SIBO can affect all of these things, and it's time to stop it.

We offer a 4-month training class called Blast Your Fat, Brain Fog, and Fatigue. This class provides you with personalized protocols based on advanced lab testing like the Great Plains Urinary OAT Test. We also track what your fungal antibodies are on the IgG immunity panel to provide personalized dietary recommendations.

What is so amazing about our program is that it finds the root cause of your SIBO, and it will lead to you feeling your best. You will be able to go at your own pace online while using customized solutions for your gut health.

If this solution is something that interests you, visit thegutinstitute.com/blast.

Whether you decide to join the program or not, I wish you good luck on your journey in overcoming SIBO and finding better and more balanced health.

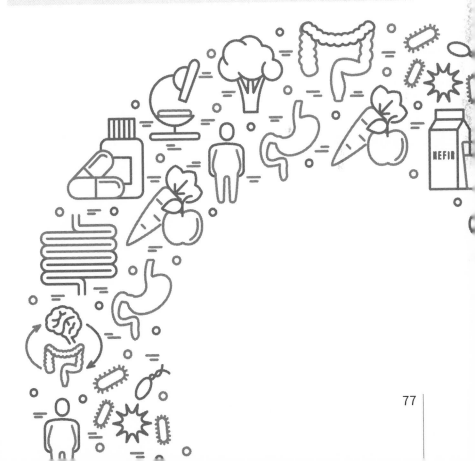

References

CHAPTER 1

Cole G.T., Seshan K.R., Lynn K.T., Franco M. Gastrointestinal candidiasis: Histopathology of candida-host interactions in a murine model. Mycol. Res. 1993;97:385–408.

Van der Waaij D., Vries J.M.B.-D., der Wees J.E.C.L.-V. Colonization resistance of the digestive tract in conventional and antibiotic-treated mice. J. Hyg. 1971;69:405–411.

Clark J.D. Influence of antibiotics or certain intestinal bacteria on orally administered candida albicans in germ-free and conventional mice. Infect. Immun. 1971;4:731–737.

Samonis G., Gikas A., Anaissie E.J., Vrenzos G., Maraki S., Tselentis Y., Bodey G.P. Prospective evaluation of effects of broad-spectrum antibiotics on gastrointestinal yeast colonization of humans. Antimicrob. Agents Chemother. 1993;37:51–53.

Pérez-Cobas A.E., Gosalbes M.J., Friedrichs A., Knecht H., Artacho A., Eismann K., Otto W., Rojo D., Bargiela R., von Bergen M., et al. Gut microbiota disturbance during antibiotic therapy: A multi-omic approach. Gut. 2013;62:1591–1601.

Dethlefsen L., Huse S., Sogin M.L., Relman D.A. The pervasive effects of an antibiotic on the human gut microbiota, as revealed by deep 16s rRNA sequencing. PLoS Biol. 2008;6:e280

Erb Downward J.R., Falkowski N.R., Mason K.L., Muraglia R., Huffnagle G.B. Modulation of post-antibiotic bacterial community reassembly and host response by candida albicans. Sci. Rep. 2013;3:2191.

Mason K.L., Erb Downward J.R., Mason K.D., Falkowski N.R., Eaton K.A., Kao J.Y., Young V.B., Huffnagle G.B. Candida albicans and bacterial microbiota interactions in the cecum during recolonization following broad-spectrum antibiotic therapy. Infect. Immun. 2012;80:3371–3380.

Mason K.L., Erb Downward J.R., Falkowski N.R., Young V.B., Kao J.Y., Huffnagle G.B. Interplay between the gastric bacterial microbiota and candida albicans during postantibiotic recolonization and gastritis. Infect. Immun. 2012;80:150–158.

Cruz M.R., Graham C.E., Gagliano B.C., Lorenz M.C., Garsin D.A. Enterococcus faecalis inhibits hyphal morphogenesis and virulence of candida albicans. Infect. Immun. 2013;81:189–200.

Scott FI, Horton DB, Mamtani R, Haynes K, Goldberg DS, Lee DY, Lewis JD. Administration of Antibiotics to Children Before Age 2 Years Increases Risk for Childhood Obesity. Gastroenterology. 2016 Jul;151(1):120-129.e5.

Bailey LC, Forrest CB, Zhang P, Richards TM, Livshits A, DeRusso PA. Association of antibiotics in infancy with early childhood obesity. JAMA Pediatr. 2014 Nov;168(11):1063-9.

Stevens V, Dumyati G, Fine LS, Fisher SG, van Wijngaarden E. Cumulative antibiotic exposures over time and the risk of Clostridium difficile infection. Clin Infect Dis. 2011 Jul 1;53(1):42-8.

Stevens V, Dumyati G, Brown J, Wijngaarden E.Differential risk of Clostridium difficile infection with proton pump inhibitor use by level of antibiotic exposure. Pharmacoepidemiol Drug Saf. 2011 Oct;20(10):1035-42.

CHAPTER 2

Sajilata, M. G., Singhal, R. S., & Kulkarni, P. R. Resistant starch – A review. Comprehensive Reviews in Food Science and Food Safety. 2006;5:1–17.

Purwani EY, Purwadaria T, Suhartono MT. Fermentation RS3 derived from sago and rice starch with Clostridium butyricum BCC B2571 or Eubacterium rectale DSM 17629. Anaerobe. 2012 Feb;18(1):55-61.

Dongowski G, Jacobasch G, Schmiedl D. Structural stability and prebiotic properties of resistant starch type 3 increase bile acid turnover and lower secondary bile acid formation. J Agric Food Chem. 2005 Nov 16;53(23):9257-67.
hole cereal grains and potential health effects: Involvement of the gut microbiota.

Gong L, Cao W, Chi H, Wang J, Zhang H, Liu J, Sun B. Whole cereal grains and potential health effects: Involvement of the gut microbiota. Food Res Int. 2018 Jan;103:84-102.

Mikulíková, D., Masár, S., & Kraic, J. Biodiversity of legume health-promoting starch. Starch. 2008;60:426–432.

CHAPTER 3

Zhong C, Qu C, Wang B, Liang S, Zeng B. Probiotics for Preventing and Treating Small Intestinal Bacterial Overgrowth: A Meta-Analysis and Systematic Review of Current Evidence. J Clin Gastroenterol. 2017 Apr;51(4):300-311.

Singhi SC, Kumar S. Probiotics in critically ill children. F1000Res. 2016 Mar 29;5.

Liang S, Xu L, Zhang D, Wu Z. Effect of probiotics on small intestinal bacterial overgrowth in patients with gastric and colorectal cancer. Turk J Gastroenterol. 2016 May;27(3):227-32.

Leventogiannis K, Gkolfakis P, Spithakis G, Tsatali A, Pistiki A, Sioulas A, Giamarellos-Bourboulis EJ, Triantafyllou K. Effect of a Preparation of Four Probiotics on Symptoms of Patients with Irritable Bowel Syndrome: Association with Intestinal Bacterial Overgrowth. Probiotics Antimicrob Proteins. 2018 Mar 5.

Chen WC, Quigley EM. Probiotics, prebiotics & synbiotics in small intestinal bacterial overgrowth: opening up a new therapeutic horizon! Indian J Med Res. 2014 Nov;140(5):582-4.

Khalighi AR, Khalighi MR, Behdani R, Jamali J, Khosravi A, Kouhestani Sh, Radmanesh H, Esmaeelzadeh S, Khalighi N. Evaluating the efficacy of probiotic on treatment in patients with small intestinal bacterial overgrowth (SIBO)--a pilot study. Indian J Med Res. 2014 Nov;140(5):604-8. [SBO probiotic Bacillus coagulans]

Gabrielli M, Lauritano EC, Scarpellini E, Lupascu A, Ojetti V, Gasbarrini G, Silveri NG, Gasbarrini A. Bacillus clausii as a treatment of small intestinal bacterial overgrowth. Am J Gastroenterol. 2009 May;104(5):1327-8. [SBO probiotic Bacillus clausii]

Bested AC, Logan AC, Selhub EM. Intestinal microbiota, probiotics and mental health: from Metchnikoff to modern advances: Part II - contemporary contextual research. Gut Pathog. 2013 Mar 14;5(1):3.

Miller AW, Oakeson KF, Dale C, Dearing MD. Microbial Community Transplant Results in Increased and Long-Term Oxalate Degradation. Microb Ecol. 2016 Aug;72(2):470-8.

Giardina S, Scilironi C, Michelotti A, Samuele A, Borella F, Daglia M,

Marzatico F. In vitro anti-inflammatory activity of selected oxalate-degrading probiotic bacteria: potential applications in the prevention and treatment of hyperoxaluria. J Food Sci. 2014 Mar;79(3):M384-90.

Al-Wahsh I, Wu Y, Liebman M. Acute probiotic ingestion reduces gastrointestinal oxalate absorption in healthy subjects. Urol Res. 2012 Jun;40(3):191-6.

Jacobs C, Coss Adame E, Attaluri A, Valestin J, Rao SS. Dysmotility and proton pump inhibitor use are independent risk factors for small intestinal bacterial and/or fungal overgrowth. Aliment Pharmacol Ther. 2013 Jun;37(11):1103-11.

Kumar S, Singhi S. Role of probiotics in prevention of Candida infection in critically ill children. Mycoses. 2013 May;56(3):204-11.

Payne S, Gibson G, Wynne A, Hudspith B, Brostoff J, Tuohy K. In vitro studies on colonization resistance of the human gut microbiota to Candida albicans and the effects of tetracycline and Lactobacillus plantarum LPK. Curr Issues Intest Microbiol. 2003 Mar;4(1):1-8.

Pärtty A, Kalliomäki M, Wacklin P, Salminen S, Isolauri E. A possible link between early probiotic intervention and the risk of neuropsychiatric disorders later in childhood: a randomized trial. Pediatr Res. 2015 Jun;77(6):823-8.

Bures J, Cyrany J, Kohoutova D, Förstl M, Rejchrt S, Kvetina J, Vorisek V, Kopacova M. Small intestinal bacterial overgrowth syndrome. World J Gastroenterol. 2010 Jun 28;16(24):2978-90.

CHAPTER 4

Salazar N, Gueimonde M, de Los Reyes-Gavilán CG, Ruas-Madiedo P. Exopolysaccharides Produced by Lactic Acid Bacteria and Bifidobacteria as Fermentable Substrates by the Intestinal Microbiota. Crit Rev Food Sci Nutr. 2016 Jul 3;56(9):1440-53.

Hutkins RW, Krumbeck JA, Bindels LB, Cani PD, Fahey G Jr, Goh YJ, Hamaker B, Martens EC, Mills DA, Rastal RA, Vaughan E, Sanders ME. Prebiotics: why definitions matter. Curr Opin Biotechnol. 2016 Feb;37:1-7.

Roberfroid M, Gibson GR, Hoyles L, McCartney AL, Rastall R, Rowland I, Wolvers D, Watzl B, Szajewska H, Stahl B, Guarner F, Respondek F, Whelan K, Coxam V, Davicco MJ, Léotoing L, Wittrant Y, Delzenne NM, Cani PD, Neyrinck AM, Meheust A. Prebiotic effects: metabolic and health benefits. Br J Nutr. 2010 Aug;104 Suppl 2:S1-63.

Petschow B, Doré J, Hibberd P, Dinan T, Reid G, Blaser M, Cani PD, Degnan FH, Foster J, Gibson G, Hutton J, Klaenhammer TR, Ley R, Nieuwdorp M, Pot B, Relman D, Serazin A, Sanders ME. Probiotics, prebiotics, and the host microbiome: the science of translation. Ann N Y Acad Sci. 2013 Dec;1306:1-17.

Firmansyah A, Chongviriyaphan N, Dillon DH, Khan NC, Morita T, Tontisirin K, Tuyen LD, Wang W, Bindels J, Deurenberg P, Ong S, Hautvast J, Meyer D, Vaughan EE. Fructans in the first 1000 days of life and beyond, and for pregnancy. Asia Pac J Clin Nutr. 2016 Dec;25(4):652-675.

Goh YJ, Klaenhammer TR. Genetic mechanisms of prebiotic oligosaccharide metabolism in probiotic microbes. Annu Rev Food Sci Technol. 2015;6:137-56.

Genta S, Cabrera W, Habib N, Pons J, Carillo IM, Grau A, Sánchez S. Yacon syrup: beneficial effects on obesity and insulin resistance in humans.

Clin Nutr. 2009 Apr;28(2):182-7. [FOS, fructo oligosaccharides]

Keithley J, Swanson B. Glucomannan and obesity: a critical review. Altern Ther Health Med. 2005 Nov-Dec;11(6):30-4.

Louis P, Flint HJ, Michel C. How to Manipulate the Microbiota: Prebiotics. Adv Exp Med Biol. 2016;902:119-42.

Van den Abbeele P, Verstraete W, El Aidy S, Geirnaert A, Van de Wiele T. Prebiotics, faecal transplants and microbial network units to stimulate biodiversity of the human gut microbiome. Microb Biotechnol. 2013 Jul;6(4):335-40.

Linares DM, Ross P, Stanton C. Beneficial Microbes: The pharmacy in the gut. Bioengineered. 2016;7(1):11-20.

CHAPTER 5

Mitchell CM, Davy BM, Hulver MW, Neilson AP, Bennett BJ, Davy KP. Does Exercise Alter Gut Microbial Composition?-A Systematic Review. Med Sci Sports Exerc. 2018 Aug 28.

Clarke SF, Murphy EF, O'Sullivan O, Lucey AJ, Humphreys M, Hogan A, Hayes P, O'Reilly M, Jeffery IB, Wood-Martin R, Kerins DM, Quigley E, Ross RP, O'Toole PW, Molloy MG, Falvey E, Shanahan F, Cotter PD. Exercise and associated dietary extremes impact on gut microbial diversity. Gut. 2014 Dec;63(12):1913-20.

Barton W, Penney NC, Cronin O, Garcia-Perez I, Molloy MG, Holmes E, Shanahan F, Cotter PD, O'Sullivan O. The microbiome of professional athletes differs from that of more sedentary subjects in composition and particularly at the functional metabolic level. Gut. 2018 Apr;67(4):625-633.

CHAPTER 6

Coucke F. Food intolerance in patients with manifest autoimmunity. Observational study. Autoimmun Rev. 2018 Sep 10. pii: S1568-9972(18)30212-X.

Karakuła-Juchnowicz H, Szachta P, Opolska A, Morylowska-Topolska J, Gałęcka M, Juchnowicz D, Krukow P, Lasik Z. The role of IgG hypersensitivity in the pathogenesis and therapy of depressive disorders. Nutr Neurosci. 2017 Feb;20(2):110-118.

Du L, Shen J, Kim JJ, He H, Chen B, Dai N. Impact of gluten consumption in patients with functional dyspepsia: A case-control study. J Gastroenterol Hepatol. 2018 Jan;33(1):128-133.

Bischoff SC, Barbara G, Buurman W, Ockhuizen T, Schulzke JD, Serino M, Tilg H, Watson A, Wells JM. Intestinal permeability--a new target for disease prevention and therapy. BMC Gastroenterol. 2014 Nov 18;14:189.

Leonard MM, Sapone A, Catassi C, Fasano A. Celiac Disease and Nonceliac Gluten Sensitivity: A Review. JAMA. 2017 Aug 15;318(7):647-656.

CHAPTER 7

Moloney RD, Desbonnet L, Clarke G, Dinan TG, Cryan JF. The microbiome: stress, health and disease. Mamm Genome. 2014 Feb;25(1-2):49-74.

Rieder R, Wisniewski PJ, Alderman BL, Campbell SC. Microbes and mental health: A review. Brain Behav Immun. 2017 Nov;66:9-17.

Cryan JF, Dinan TG. Mind-altering microorganisms: the impact of the gut microbiota on brain and behaviour. Nat Rev Neurosci. 2012 Oct;13(10):701-12.

Zhao TT, Shin KS, Choi HS, Lee MK. Ameliorating effects of gypenosides on chronic stress-induced anxiety disorders in mice. BMC Complement Altern Med. 2015 Sep 14;15:323. [Gynostemma pentophyllum, anticancer, adaptogen]

Chen L, Brar MS, Leung FC, Hsiao WL. Triterpenoid herbal saponins enhance beneficial bacteria, decrease sulfate-reducing bacteria, modulate inflammatory intestinal microenvironment and exert cancer preventive effects in ApcMin/+ mice. Oncotarget. 2016 May 24;7(21):31226-42. [Gynostemma pentophyllum, anticancer, adaptogen]

Liu J, Li Y, Yang P, Wan J, Chang Q, Wang TTY, Lu W, Zhang Y, Wang Q, Yu LL. Gypenosides Reduced the Risk of Overweight and Insulin Resistance in C57BL/6J Mice through Modulating Adipose Thermogenesis and Gut Microbiota. J Agric Food Chem. 2017 Oct 25;65(42):9237-9246. [Gynostemma pentophyllum, anticancer, adaptogen, raises probiotic Akkermansia]

Novik GI, Astapovich NI, Riabaia NE, Bogdan AS. [Biological activity of the protein-polysaccharide complex secreted by Bifidobacterium adolescentis]. Mikrobiologiia. 1997 Sep-Oct;66(5):628-34.

Jin M, Zhu Y, Shao D, Zhao K, Xu C, Li Q, Yang H, Huang Q, Shi J. Effects of polysaccharide from mycelia of Ganoderma lucidum on intestinal barrier functions of rats. Int J Biol Macromol. 2017 Jan;94(Pt A):1-9. [Reishi Ganoderma lucidum raised sIgA, microbiome diversity and intestinal barrier function]

Li K, Zhuo C, Teng C, Yu S, Wang X, Hu Y, Ren G, Yu M, Qu J. Effects of Ganoderma lucidum polysaccharides on chronic pancreatitis and intestinal microbiota in mice. Int J Biol Macromol. 2016 Dec;93(Pt A):904-912. [Reishi Ganoderma lucidum raised diversity, Lactobacilli, Roseburia and Lachnospiraceae, raised SOD, resolved pancreatitis, lowered lipases, AMS, IFN-γ and TNF-α]

Chang CJ, Lin CS, Lu CC, Martel J, Ko YF, Ojcius DM, Tseng SF, Wu TR, Chen YY, Young JD, Lai HC. Ganoderma lucidum reduces obesity in mice by modulating the composition of the gut microbiota. Nat Commun. 2015 Jun 23;6:7489. [Mice: Reishi Ganoderma lucidum reduced endotoxin-bearing Proteobacteria levels, improved intestinal barrier integrity, metabolic endotoxemia, reversed insulin resistance, induced weight loss and reduce inflammation]

Yang Y, Nirmagustina DE, Kumrungsee T, Okazaki Y, Tomotake H, Kato N. Feeding of the water extract from Ganoderma lingzhi to rats modulates secondary bile acids, intestinal microflora, mucins, and propionate important to colon cancer. Biosci Biotechnol Biochem. 2017 Sep;81(9):1796-1804. [Reishi Ganoderma lingzhi increases sIgA, mucin and decreased Clostridium]